E00876

AF835544

THE BRISTOL MEDICAL SCHOOL

May I first of all express my thanks to the University of Bristol for inviting me to give this lecture in honour of an enthusiastic historian of Bristol, Frederick Creech Jones. A photograph of him taken about 1920 on the base of the Whitchurch Cross illustrates his interest in antiquities (see p. 2). His working life was spent with the Bristol Waterworks Company whose history he wrote on the occasion of their centenary in 1946. In the same year he published his book *The Glory that was Bristol* in which he recorded many historical Bristol buildings and deplored the loss of so many of them not only by enemy action but also by urban 'development' in the period before the war. The losses included the Barber Surgeons' Hall in Shannon Court. I think therefore that Mr Creech Jones might have approved the subject of my lecture.

Regular medical training may be held to have started in Bristol on 20 June 1737 when the Infirmary first opened its doors to patients. From the start the Apothecary – the resident general practitioner – was allowed apprentices, and shortly afterwards surgical apprentices were admitted as well. In the first half of the eighteenth century, anyone who wished could practice medicine without necessarily having any qualification or experience. However, the more regular practitioners fell into four groups. First, there were the Apothecaries who carried out most of what we now call general practice. They had separated from the Grocers' Company in the previous century but served a seven years apprenticeship. There were about thirty in Bristol at that time, and although they

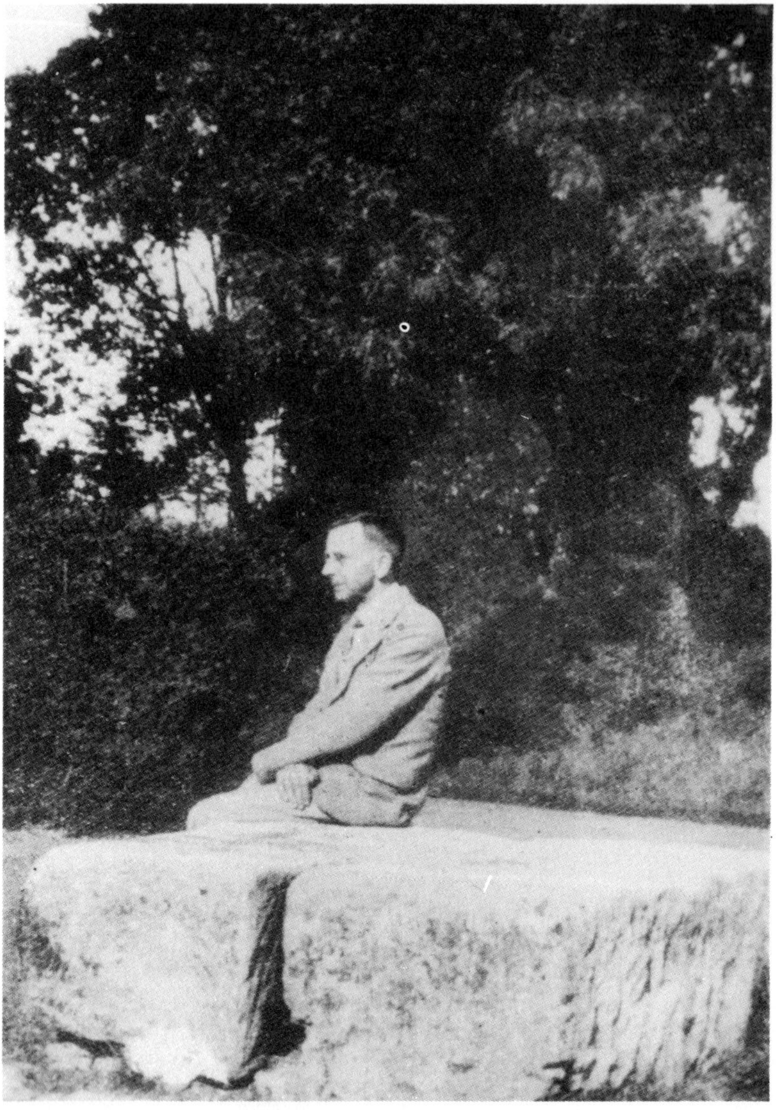

Mr. F.C. Jones c. 1920

were allowed to charge only for medicines and not for advice, the medicines were dispensed in such large amounts that some of them acquired a very lucrative practice. One of the more successful apothecaries is said to have made over £4,000 a year.

Then, there were the Barber Surgeons and the Surgeons. They were gradually parting company and the two guilds finally separated in 1745. At this time there were in the City about twelve Barber Surgeons and twenty Surgeons. They, too, were trained by a seven years apprenticeship and treated fractures and injuries, bled patients at the request of the Physicians and cut for the stone. The last Barber Surgeon to practice in Bristol had his sign next to the Guildhall in Broad Street and died in 1807. He was said to have dressed more wigs, drawn more teeth and shed more blood than any man in Bristol.

Then there were the Physicians of whom there were five or six in Bristol. They were graduates of Oxford, Cambridge, Edinburgh or St. Andrew's or of a foreign University like Padua or Montpellier. It was said that they had a good knowledge of the classics and held their heads high. They might graduate knowing all the writings of Galen, but without necessarily seeing a patient. Not all Universities were particular about their requirements for the M.D. As late as 1792 when Edward Jenner, the discoverer of vaccination, who had been apprenticed to Mr. Ludlow, a surgeon, at Sodbury and then studied at St. George's Hospital, thought he would like to practice as a physician in Cheltenham during the season, St. Andrew's agreed to confer the degree of Doctor of Medicine on him upon the recommendation of Dr. Hicks of Gloucester and Dr. Parry of Bath. Admittedly by then he was already a Fellow of the Royal Society, but that was for his observations on the cuckoo.

Physicians in the early part of the century were very particular as to dress. It is recorded that Dr. Logan, one of the first Infirmary Physicians, never appeared in the wards unless in full professional dress – his head covered with an immense flowing wig, a red roquelaure hanging from his shoulders to his heels, his wrist graced with a gold headed cane, and his side furnished with a long French rapier. It would appear that ward rounds must have been far more impressive then than they are now.

Another physician on the staff of the Infirmary in the middle of the eighteenth century was Dr. Lyne, who earned a great reputation with a secret cure for dropsy. It finally transpired that this was Bristol Milk. His practice clearly flourished, as after eight years on the staff he resigned with a letter which must be nearly a record for

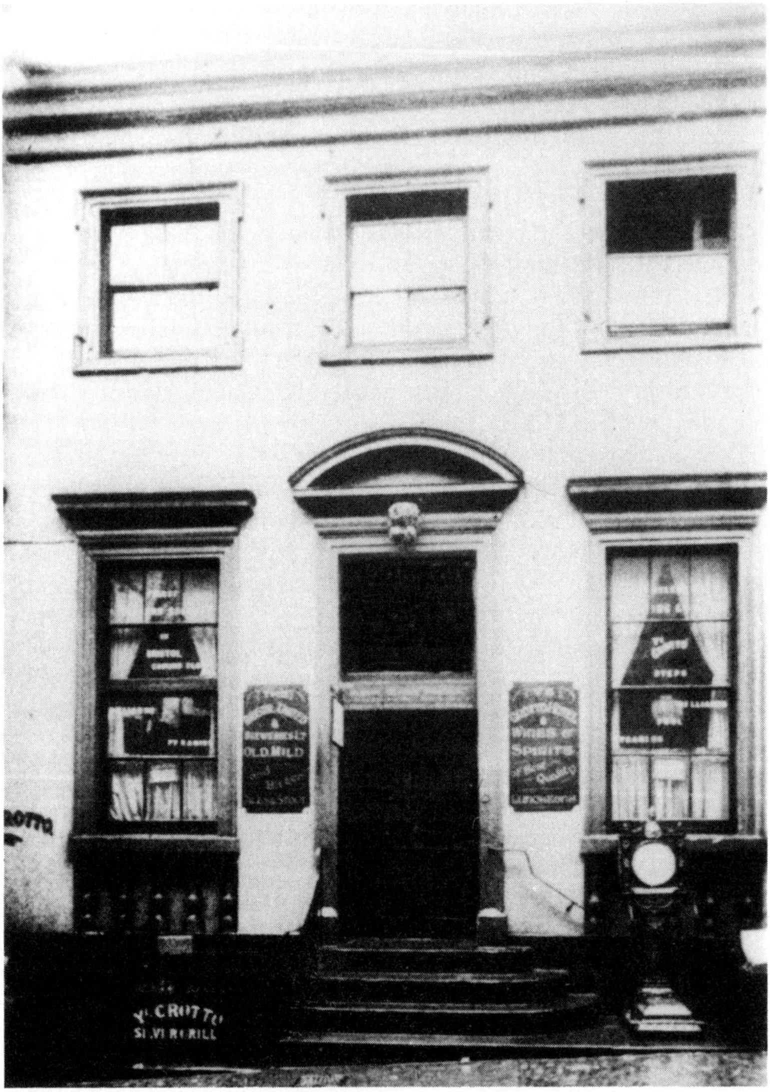

The Barber Surgeons' Hall, later the West Indian Coffee House and then The Grapes Public House

brevity:– 'Gentlemen, the Infirmary interferes so much with my private affairs that I cannot possibly attend to all. I therefore resign and am, Gentlemen, your humble servant. Edward Lyne.'

Towards the end of the century a more distinguished physician at the Infirmary was Dr. Edward Long Fox senior, who was one of the first to take a humane view of lunacy and built Brislington House as a private asylum. His reputation was such that he was called to Windsor in consultation on George III.

A notable surgeon at about the same time was Richard Smith junior. He was a great magpie and collected not only pathological specimens – forming a most valuable teaching museum – but also letters, reports, press cuttings, advertisements, and everything in any way connected with the Infirmary. These are now bound and deposited in the City Archives where they constitute an inexhaustible source of material for historians both of the Infirmary and of the City.

Throughout the eighteenth century the Infirmary was steadily enlarged so that by 1752 there were 150 beds. Forty years later a rebuilding took place which resulted in what we still know as the 'old building'. With these expansions there was ample provision for clinical teaching of students who also attended St. Peter's Hospital and the Clifton Dispensary and it was natural that courses of lectures, particularly on Anatomy – then the only pre-clinical science – should be organised. These were advertised in the local press and open to the public. One of the first of these was given by Drs. Page and Ford in the anatomical theatre of the Barber Surgeons' Hall in 1744. Fifteen years later Ford resigned as surgeon to the Infirmary and moved to London where he was appointed Physician Accoucheur to Queen Charlotte. It is said that he lost a lot of money when, with Richard Brinsley Sheridan, he bought David Garrick's share of Drury Lane Theatre. The Barber Surgeons' Hall built in 1690 off Exchange Avenue survived until destroyed this century. With the dissolution of the Guild in 1745 it became the West Indian Coffee House and finally a public house known as The Grapes with a restaurant on the ground floor.

Similar short-lived courses of lectures were instituted by Mr. Godfrey Lowe in 1756 and another by Mr. Miller in Terrell Street in 1785.

A more ambitious project of Anatomy lectures was organised in 1797 at the Red Lodge by Drs. Beddoes, Bowles and Smith. These attracted large audiences, but the introductory lecture nearly came to grief. Beddoes promised to write it for Bowles to

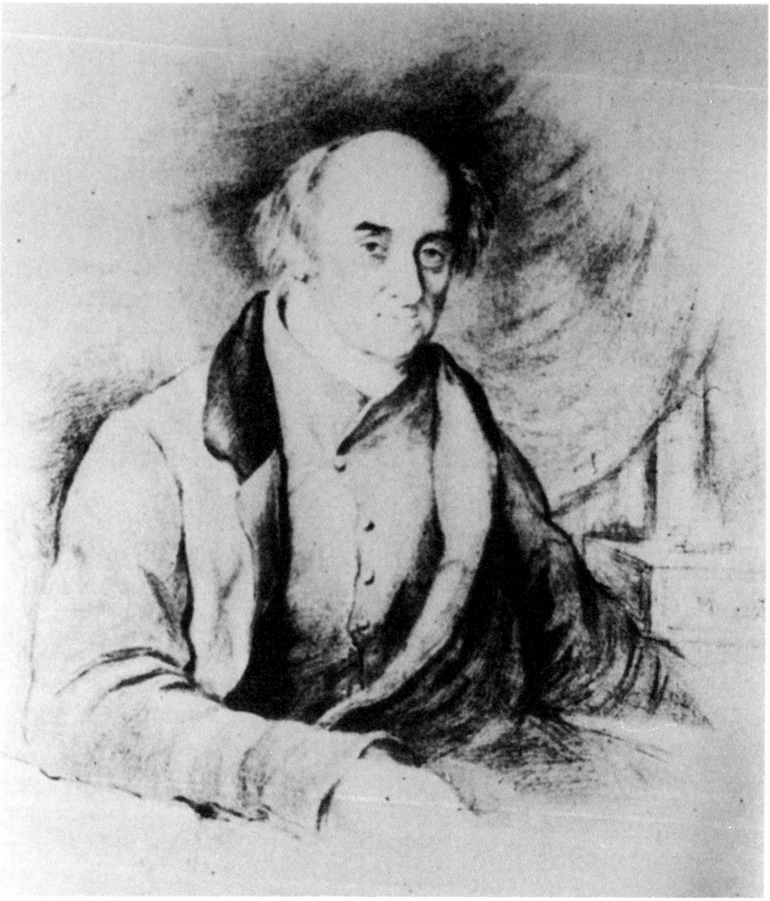

Edward Long Fox Senior

read, but he was so dilatory in preparing it that it only arrived half an hour after the lecture was due to start, having been brought by Bowles completely out of breath having run all the way from Clifton. Even so, he had great difficulty in reading it as the text was nearly illegible. Beddoes had been a lecturer in Chemistry at Oxford, but left under a cloud, having shown too great enthusiasm for and support for the French revolutionaries. He came to Bristol, but he never succeeded in being elected to the staff of the Infirmary. He established the Pneumatick Institute in Dowry Square where he advocated the use of various gases, or factitious airs, in therapy. It is said that he even went so far as to recommend the inhalation of a cow's breath for consumption. The main importance of the Pneumatick Institute is that at the age of 21 Humphrey Davy was appointed superintendent and here experimented with the effects of 'laughing gas' – nitrous oxide – on himself, Coleridge, Southey and others, including 'various lady friends'. He foretold its probable use in surgery. It is surprising and fortunate that no tragedy occurred at these sessions. It is probable that the recipients of the gas also had access to plenty of oxygen in the air owing to the rather primitive apparatus.

In 1800 the College of Surgeons received its Charter, and its examinations, although optional, became popular. The College required students to produce evidence of attendance at lectures and classes. This led to the institution of further schools. In 1807 Mr. White built dissecting rooms in Limekiln Lane, Lower College Street – the site is now covered by a large garage – and lectured regularly until his death in 1816. The school was carried on by Dr. Wallis, who later enlisted the help of others. In 1822 it moved to Lamb Street, Bishop's Park, and became known as the Bristol School of Anatomy and Medicine. These lectures were recognised by the College of Surgeons.

In 1813 Francis Gold, who had been interned in France as a result of the war but who was released by Napolean at the request of Edward Jenner, lectured on Anatomy and Physiology at 3 College Green, close to the Cathedral cloisters. The site is now covered by the nave of the Cathedral and some say that the Cathedral pulpit stands on the site of the anatomy lecture theatre. In 1819 Gold joined the Indian Medical Service, but the lectures were carried on by Dr. Goodeve until 1827. In 1814 Dr. James Cowles Prichard, a famous anthropologist and physician at the Infirmary, organised lectures on Physiology, Pathology, and the Practice of Medicine, at his house in College Green. Later he was

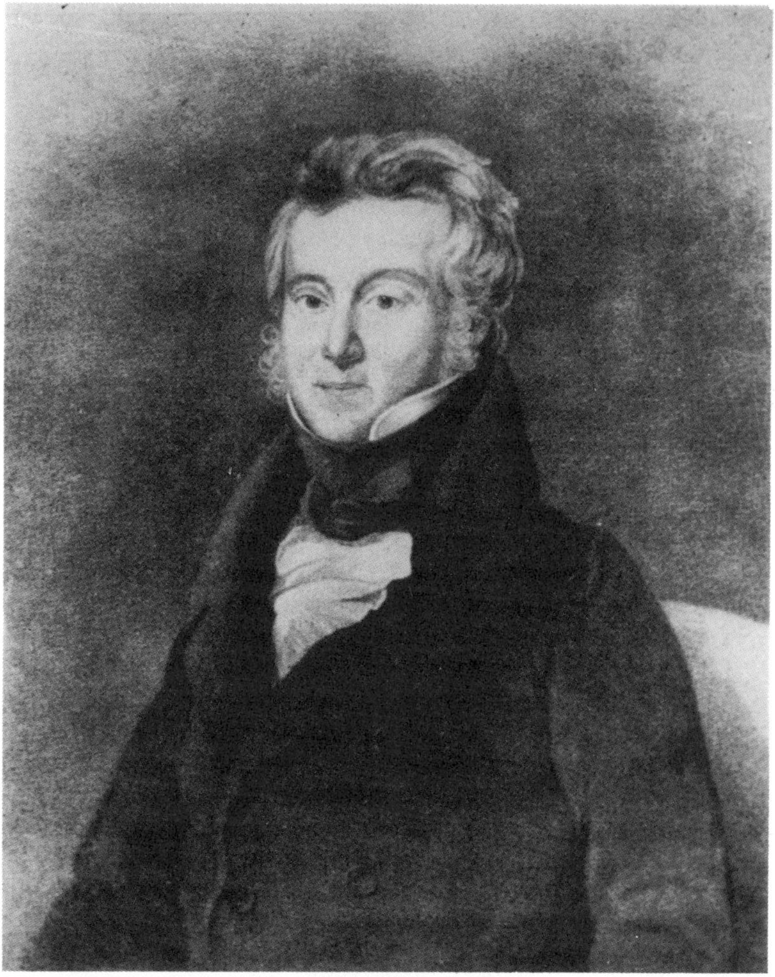
Dr. Richard Smith junior

very active in the formation of Bristol College and became a member of its Council.

A further impetus to more organised medical training came from the Society of Apothecaries when in 1815 they were authorized to prosecute unqualified apothecaries and to examine and licence all new men. In 1826 Mr. Henry Clark established what he called the Bristol Medical and Surgical School at 3 King's Square. His lectures were recognised by the Society of Apothecaries in 1828.

In 1831, since the Infirmary was unable to deal with all the patients coming to it, a Committee was formed, many members of which belonged to the Society of Friends, to establish the General Hospital, which opened in Guinea Street in 1832. At the opening ceremony it was stated that the Committee had no doubt that the Establishment would become a useful school of Medical Instruction. Progress was at first slow owing to financial difficulties, but things improved, and in 1858 a new hospital, built near the Guinea Street site, was opened. Following this there was a steady expansion by new buildings. Until they amalgamated in 1940, the Infirmary and Hospital existed in not always friendly rivalry. The Infirmary was largely supported by Church and Tories and the Hospital by Nonconformists and Whigs. Hence the saying that patients going to the Infirmary could expect a sovereign remedy, while those going to the Hospital would receive a radical cure.

In 1833 the lecturers from most of the various schools, with the exception of Wallis, combined with some of the staff of the Infirmary and of the new General Hospital, to establish the Bristol Medical School. This was initially housed in the premises of Mr. Clark in King's Square. In the inaugural lecture given by Dr. Carrick, the Senior Physician at the Infirmary, the hope was expressed that the School of Medicine might become an integral part of Bristol College. Founded in 1831, this taught Classics and Mathematics and appeared to be flourishing. At first this idea was favourably received, but finally the Council of the College decided 'that it was not expedient to recommend the union'. This may have been because the Medical School insisted on two conditions – one, a promise of adequate accommodation within a short space of time, and second, that the School should be managed by a Senatus Medicus composed of equal numbers of members of the College Council and Medical School lecturers. This may have been just as well for the Medical School. The Bristol College exhibited too liberal a character for the age and was attacked as a godless

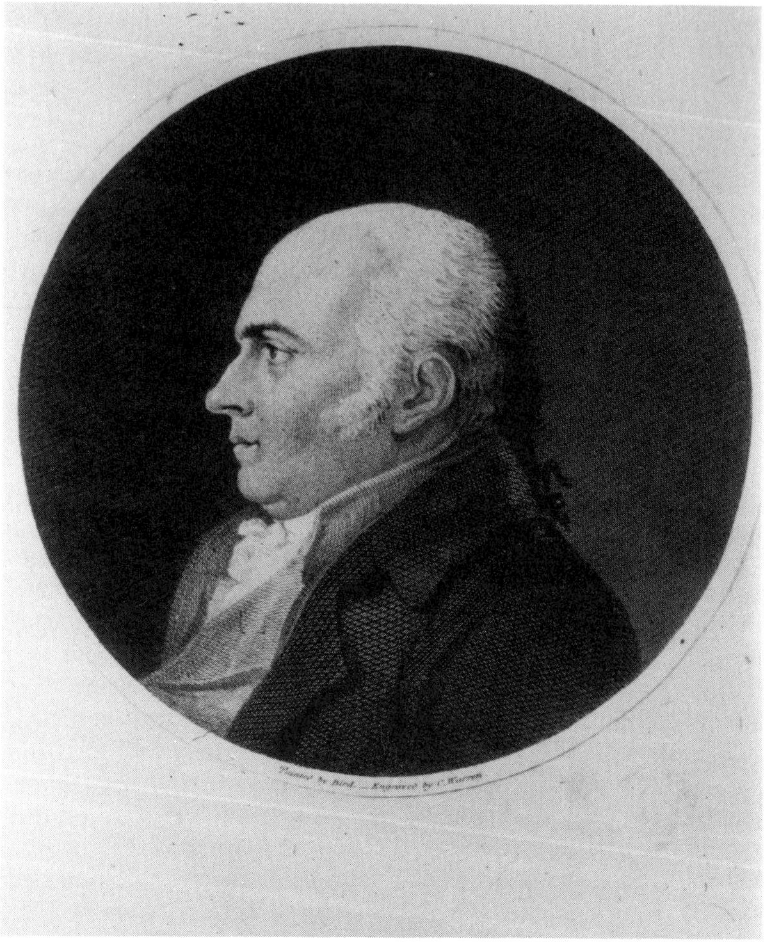

Dr. Thomas Beddoes

institution on the grounds that it failed to exclude dissenters. A rival, the Bishop's College, was founded in 1840, and the Bristol College closed its doors in 1842. However, the Bishop's College too had a fairly short life, closing in 1861.

A little mystery surrounds the badge of the Schola Medicinae Bristol as it carries the date 1828 (see front cover). This is probably because lectures given in Bristol were first recognised by the Society of Apothecaries at that date.

Initially the College of Surgeons required all candidates at their examination to have spent at least twelve months attending lectures and classes at a London hospital or at hospitals in certain Scottish and Irish cities. The Society of Apothecaries insisted on the same requirement until 1829 when they put London and provincial hospitals on the same footing and the surgeons reduced their required residence to six months. The members of the Bristol Medical School much resented this, and when in 1833 a Committee on Medical Education was appointed they sent a letter, apparently drafted by Dr. J. Addington Symonds, objecting to this requirement. One reason they gave was:– 'Vast numbers of promising young men have had their characters, their usefulness and their peace of mind irreparably ruined by even a brief sojourn in the capital where practices of immorality and licentiousness may be pursued with such great facility and so little immediate disgrace.' The requirement was rescinded in 1834.

In the same year the Medical School moved to new premises which they rented in Old Park behind the building now known as Lunsford House. At that time Lunsford House was used as a school and at times the work of the Medical School was embarrassed by noise created by its pupils, who also tried to see what was going on in the Medical School. The anatomy lecture theatre and the dissecting room survived, being used by the University Clerk of Works until destroyed by a bomb in 1941.

In its new quarters the Medical School flourished and two years later had 52 students, being the third largest provincial school after Manchester and Birmingham. In 1839 Bristol students were declared eligible to enter the examinations for the degrees in Medicine in the new University of London. The first Bristol student to take advantage of this did so in 1842.

The syllabus of the first year of the Medical School shows that the lecturers must have worked very hard. Dr. Henry Riley, for instance, undertook two courses on Anatomy and Physiology, took part in anatomical demonstrations and lectured on the whole

PROSPECTUS
ISSUED BY THE BRISTOL MEDICAL SCHOOL IN 1833.

LECTURES AT BRISTOL MEDICAL SCHOOL.

	TIME	TERMS	
		Single Course	*Unlimited*
ANATOMY AND PHYSIOLOGY, by HENRY RILEY, M.D.; *Physician to St. Peter's Hospital; and* Mr. H. CLARK, M.R.C.S.	*October to April*	£4 4 0	£8 8 0
PRINCIPLES AND PRACTICE OF SURGERY, by Mr. HETLING, M.R.C.S.; *Surgeon to the Bristol Infirmary*.	*December to June*	£3 3 0	£5 5 0
CHEMISTRY, by Mr. W. HERAPATH.	*November to April*	£3 3 0	£6 6 0
MATERIA MEDICA AND THERAPEUTICS, by Mr. G. D. FRIPP, M.R.C.S.; *Surgeon to the Bristol General Hospital.*	*January to April*	£3 3 0	£5 5 0
THEORY AND PRACTICE OF MEDICINE, by HENRY RILEY, M.D.	*April to June*	£3 3 0	£5 5 0
MIDWIFERY AND DISEASES OF WOMEN AND CHILDREN, by Mr. J. C. SWAYNE, M.R.C.S.; *Senior Consulting Accoucheur to the Bristol Dispensary.*	*January to April*	£3 3 0	£5 5 0
FORENSIC MEDICINE, by J. A. SYMONDS, M.D.; *Physician to the Bristol General Hospital.* CHEMICAL TOXICOLOGY, by Mr. W. HERAPATH.	*April to June*	£3 3 0	£5 5 0
ANATOMICAL DEMONSTRATIONS, by HENRY RILEY, M.D., and Mr. H. CLARK, M.R.C.S. ..	*November to April*	£3 3 0	£6 6 0
BOTANY, by Mr. S. ROOTSEY, F.L.S. ..	*April to June*	£3 3 0	£5 5 0

The Hours for the various Lectures will be so arranged as not to interfere with each other. *September 12th*, 1833.

theory and practice of medicine. At this time Dr. Riley was Physician to St. Peter's Hospital, which had been opened by the Guardians of the Poor as a workhouse hospital in 1698 with Dr. Dover at the first Physician. The latter achieved notoriety as a privateer and lasting fame as the inventor of Dover's powder, which in the pre-aspirin days was the popular treatment of colds and minor infections. The building survived as the offices of the Guardians until destroyed in one of the Bristol raids. It had been built as the town mansion of the Aldworth family, had been used as a sugar refinery and for two years before becoming a hospital had housed the local mint. Appointment to St. Peter's Hospital was often a stepping stone to election to the Infirmary staff and Dr. Riley duly became Physician to the Infirmary in 1834.

It is interesting to see how sometimes the same names crop up repeatedly in the history of the Medical School and of medicine in Bristol. Mr. J.S. Swayne lectured in midwifery in 1833. His son, J.G. Swayne, succeeded him in 1850 and in 1902 Walter Swayne, a nephew, was appointed Professor of Obstetrics in University College. Similarly Mr. Herapath, who lectured in Chemistry from 1833 to 1867, had a son who became an even more famous chemist and a Fellow of the Royal Society. His son was in practice in Bristol in the early years of this century and his grandson was the first cardiologist at the Infirmary. His son is now in practice at Keynsham.

J. Addington Symonds, who lectured on Forensic Medicine, was the first Physician appointed to the General Hospital and was one of the most ardent advocates of a combined Medical School. He ran a very successful practice in Berkeley Square and was so busy with this that he resigned from the Hospital in 1843 and moved to Clifton Hill House. One of his daughters married Sir Edward Strachey and was the mother of St. Loe Strachey of *Spectator* fame. His son, John Addington Symonds junior, was the famous Victorian author and critic who wrote the seven volume work on the Renaissance in Italy.

The members of the early Medical School were certainly highly dedicated. The overhead expenses of the School absorbed well over half the fees, and with fluctuating numbers of students, there was often little left to be divided amongst the lecturers, one of whom complained that his fees one year for a whole course came to 18 pence. They certainly believed in the value of lectures. Mr. Crosby Leonard, who entered the School as a student in 1845, in later life recalled that he was required to attend 140 lectures on

Descriptive and Surgical Anatomy a year for three years, the same number on General Anatomy and Physiology, and 100 lectures on each of Medicine, Surgery, Chemistry and Materia Medica. However, the clinical side of the students' work was not neglected. In 1837 the Medical School requested the Infirmary to admit an increased number of students. Each physician and each surgeon, it was agreed, should have up to six students attached to him. Further, the surgical dressers, as they were called, were to live in free of charge in turns for a week at a time, and were not allowed to leave the building until the next in turn had taken his place. During this time they were expected to see all casualties and emergencies day and night. Obviously this was a most valuable experience.

In 1860 pupils of the Pharmaceutical Society were admitted to some of the classes and a year later lectures for dental students were organised and a few years later Dental Surgeons at the Infirmary and Hospital were reognised as teachers by the Royal College of Surgeons.

In 1862 the premises used by the School were purchased by Miss Carpenter, who however renewed the lease till 1867 and then agreed to continue it on a temporary basis. But the accommodation in Old Park was becoming inadquate and in 1873 a meeting was called to organise an appeal for funds for a new building. However at this meeting Mr. Coomber, the lecturer in Chemistry, suggested that instead the Medical School should seek the co-operation of the authorities of the Museum and Library in a joint effort to establish a College of Science of which the Medical School should be a Department. The Council of the Museum and Library received this proposal very favourably and a joint Committee was formed. A great deal of support was forthcoming, especially from Prebendary Percival, the Headmaster of Clifton College. The scheme went ahead fairly quickly with promises of financial support from various sources, including £1,000 from the Medical School. There then followed much discussion as to whether the Medical School should be affiliated to, or incorporated in, the new University College. Finally agreement was reached on affiliation with the Medical School remaining autonomous but to have two members on the governing body of the College, but the School made new buildings part of the agreement. However, soon after University College opened in 1876 the Medical School ran into trouble. The staff of the Royal Infirmary were concerned at the poor results of Bristol students in the examinations of the Royal College of Surgeons. They sent a letter to the Surgeons suggesting that before any more Bristol students were admitted to the examinations the School should be inspected. The General Hospital staff refused to be associated with these complaints, but the *Lancet* took the matter up in editorials. However, the Surgeons decided that they would take no action in view of the 'transitional state' of the Medical School. Dissatisfied with this, some members of the Infirmary staff suggested forming a new rival Medical School. Finally the Medical School agreed to a new scheme for the management of the School. This reassured the Council of University College which had been reluctant to provide buildings for a school in such disarray. In 1879 affiliation with the College was agreed, the College promising to provide new buildings as soon as financially possible, but in the meantime to build a temporary brick building, the first building to be erected on the newly acquired Tyndall's Park estate. This was occupied by the Medical School in 1880. Described as a 'wretched brick shed' and a 'hideous blot on the College', it is still in existence, over 100 years later, although now screened by the permanent building erected for the Medical School financed by a public subscription largely supported by local practitioners. This building was opened in November 1892 by Sir Andrew Clarke, the President of the General Medical Council. The whole of this complex, including the temporary brick shed, is now occupied by the Department of Geography. All that remains to show its original purpose is the motto of the Royal College of Physicians over the entrance. This is the Hippocratic aphorism ὁ βίος βραχύς ἡ δὲ τεχνη μακρή translated by Chaucer 'The life so short, the craft so long to learn.'[1]

At about the same time, after a further nine years of negotiation, the Medical School became fully incorporated with, and the second faculty of, University College.

Meanwhile the Medical Act of 1858 restricted the practice of medicine to those who had passed a recognised examination and the 1886 amendment ended the so-called half qualfication by which a candidate could qualify as an apothecary or surgeon by laying down that no person should be admitted to the medical register who had not passed an examination in medicine, surgery and midwifery – hence the conjoint board.

In the latter part of the nineteenth century there were a number

1. *The Parliament of Fowls.*

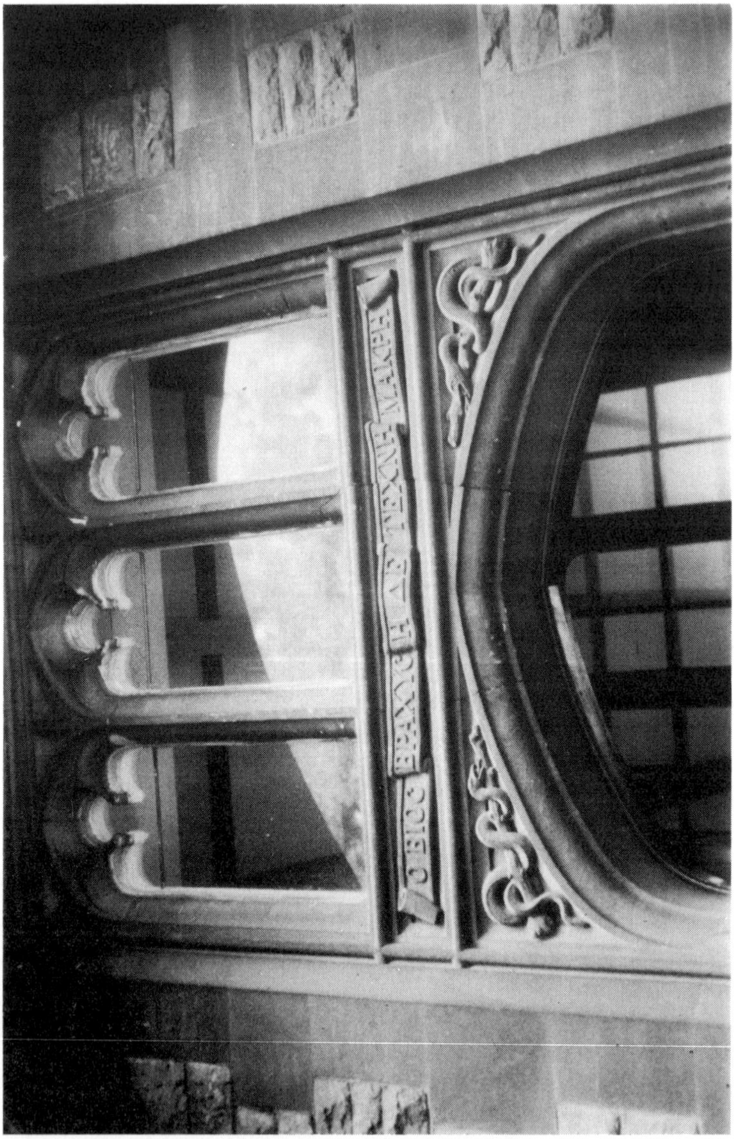

The first University Medical School

of prominent members of the Medical School. William Budd – Physician to the Infirmary from 1847 to 1862 – is often called the father of epidemiology. Long before any causal bacterium had been discovered he described how typhoid fever and cholera probably spread by water. This made him, as described by Mr. Creech Jones, a most valuable and active member of the first Council of the Bristol Waterworks Company. Again before the tubercle bacillus had been found he argued that phthisis was contagious. He described how he came to this conclusion, which was fiercely attacked by some of his Bristol colleagues, as follows:–

'The idea that phthisis is a self propagating disease and that all the leading phenomenon of its distribution may be explained by supposing that it is disseminated through society by specific germs cast off by persons already suffering from the disease first came to mind, unbidden so to speak, while I was walking on the Observatory Hill at Clifton in the second week in August 1856.'

Far from rushing into print he waited seven years before publishing this idea. Incidentally his brother, Francis Nonus Budd, was the first Chairman of Council of University College 1876–1882.

Budd's successor as Physician to the Infirmary was John Beddoe. He achieved worldwide fame as a physical anthropologist and wrote a book on the *Races of Britain*. When the British Association met in Bristol in 1875 he was invited to be President of the anthropological section, but he declined, explaining that 'I could not afford to let my scientific reputation injure my medical practice.'

In 1930 when the British Association were again meeting in Bristol, Sir Arthur Keith in a Beddoe memorial lecture said:–

'We owe more to him than to any other anthropologist of the Victorian epoch.' He went on to urge the University to found a chair of anthropology in his memory. Sadly this has still to be achieved.

A student of considerable distinction entered the Medical School in 1869. At the age of seventeen he had already scored a century when playing for England. W.G. Grace did not qualify until ten years later and then via Barts and Westminster.

Edward Long Fox junior, the grandson of the founder of Brislington House, graduated M.B. Oxford in 1857 and the same year was appointed Physician to the Infirmary. He became a well-known neurologist and was Bradshaw lecturer at the College of Physicians in 1882. He was very interested in and popular with

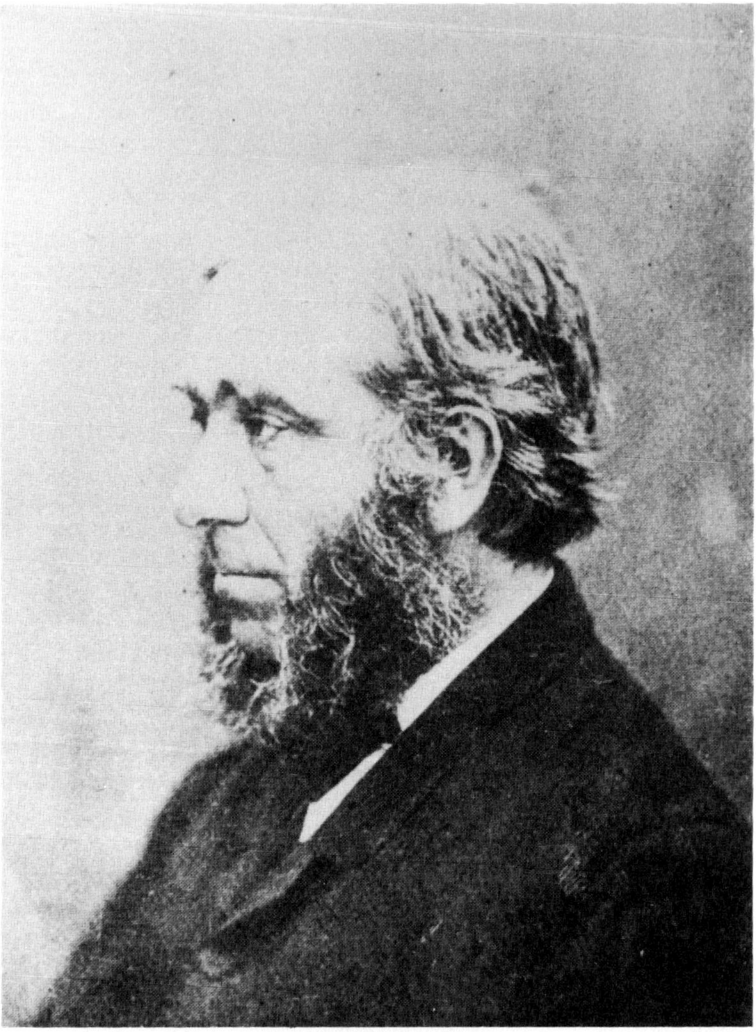

Dr. William Budd

the students, all of whom were invited to a strawberry tea party every year at his house in Clifton.

Greig Smith, Surgeon to the Infirmary from 1879–1897, was one of the pioneers of abdominal surgery. He died at the early age of 43, but his book on Abdominal Surgery ran into five editions and was translated into French. In 1893 the first full-time Professor in the Faculty of Medicine was appointed. Professor Edward Fawcett held the Chair of Anatomy for forty-one years and for the last twenty five of these was Dean of the Faculty of Medicine. For very many he personified the Bristol Medical School. His research was almost confined to vertebrate embryology for which he was elected to the Fellowship of the Royal Society.

In 1906 University College was able to announce with some pleasure that after negotiations with the Royal Infirmary and General Hospital clinical instruction had been made available to women 'who are thus provided in Bristol with the means of full preparation for the medical profession.'

When the University received its Charter in 1909 Dr. Michell Clarke, Physician to the General Hospital and one of the Professors of Medicine, was appointed the first Pro-Vice-Chancellor, an office which he held until his death in 1918. This may have been in recognition of the part played by the Medical School in the development of University College.

Following the establishment of the University, the Royal Infirmary and the General Hospital were formally recognised for clinical instruction. In addition, the Royal Hospital for Sick Children, the Eye Hospital, Ham Green Fever Hospital and the Lunatic Asylum at Fishponds were recognised for special instruction. Despite this, clinical teaching lacked complete integration with the University. Until 1922 students when embarking on clinical work paid tuition fees not to the University, but to the Hospital to which they were attached. These were then divided amongst the staff. This led to much competition between the Infirmary and Hospital to attract students. Finally it was agreed that all fees should be paid to the University and the clinical teachers were given part time University appointments and received an honorarium.

The 1892 building for the Medical School and for which it had waited for so long contained a large room housing the Medical Library and the faculty was not very pleased when in 1911 this room was taken over by the University as a Council Chamber and Senate Room. The Medical Library was then banished for four

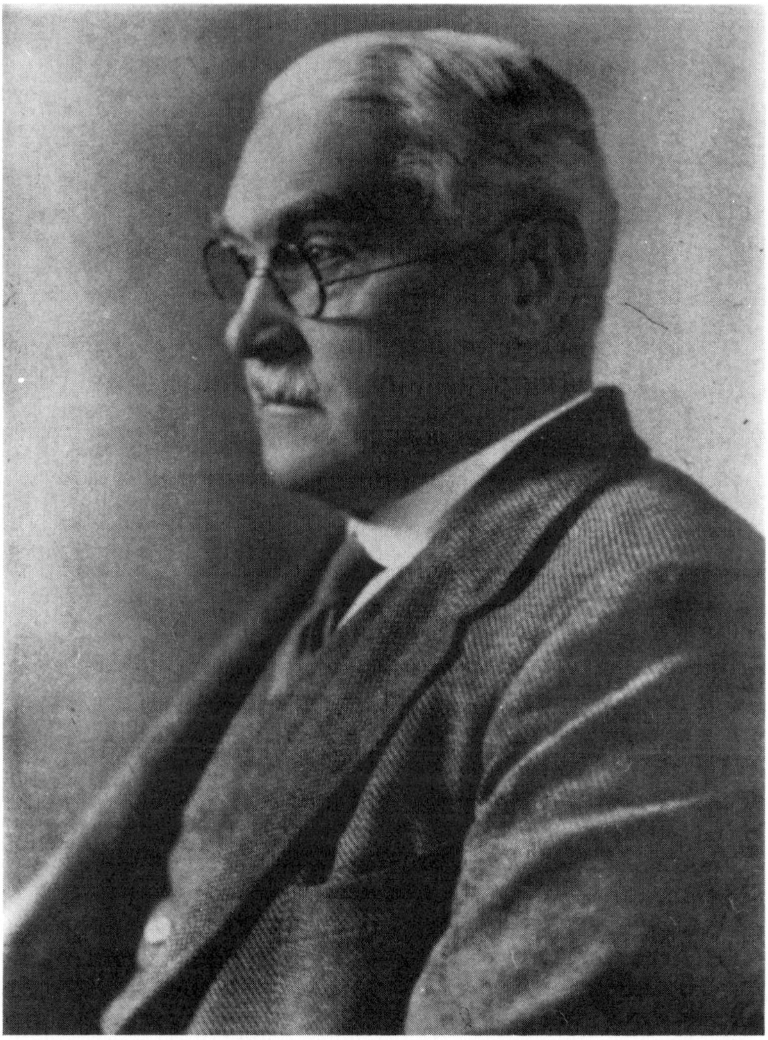

Professor Edward Fawcett, the first full-time Professor in the Faculty of Medicine, appointed in 1893

years to the basement of the old Blind Asylum and then moved again to the racquet court of the Drill Hall. There it remained till 1925, when it moved to the specially built accommodation under the main library in the Wills Memorial Building. Now, of course, it is housed in considerable style in the new Medical School. The local Medical Society, in recognition of its gift of its library to University college, was allowed to use the library for meetings, but this privilege was terminated when the Vice-Chancellor banned the use of the oxy-hydrogen lantern used for projecting slides because of the danger of fire. It was over seventy years later that the fire occurred, and then it was not due to the Society's lantern.

By the 1920's the ground floor of the Medical School had been completely taken over for University administration and a senior common room, except for the room on the right of the entrance which remained the office of the Dean of the Faculty of Medicine. The pre-clinical departments shared with the science faculty the buildings which had sprung up around the quadrangle in University Road.

In 1919 the Board of Education, perhaps stimulated by the Flexner report, wished to improve the standard of medical education. Sir George Newman, the Medical Secretary of the Board, came to Bristol and addressed a meeting of representatives of various medical charities and of the University. He told them that Bristol might have a medical school which 'was great in tradition and in the length of its history, but it was not great in all respects . . . it was' he said 'all at sixes and sevens.' He urged the co-ordination of the hospitals used for teaching into one University hospital. A medical charities committee was set up to consider this. Mr. Henry Wills, who had been convinced of the wisdom of this union, put just over £100,000 in trust for the hospitals if they amalgamated before the end of 1920. Failing this, the money was to go to the Infirmary absolutely. The Committee of the General Hospital refused to agree to the proposals and so the Infirmary received the money.

In 1925, anxious to improve clinical teaching and research, the University invited Sir Berkeley Moynihan, later Lord Moynihan, the President of the Royal College of Surgeons, to report on the best method of achieving this. He recommended that an understanding should be reached between the Royal Infirmary and General Hospital to secure a re-arrangement of patients and a fusion of the staffs and that full-time clinical professors should be appointed with adequate clinical and laboratory assistance provided by the University and that each professor should have charge of from 50 to 100 beds. After deliberation, the University decided that this report could only be implemented if the Royal Infirmary and General Hospital became branches of a single hospital. It was another fourteen years before this was agreed and the redistribution of beds and the fusion of the staffs recommended in the Moynihan report took place on 1 June 1940.

However the University persevered with its idea of full time clinical professors. It had approached the University Grants Committee for financial help in 1920, but had received the reply that while the University Grants Committee approved the scheme, it offered no hope of an increased grant. Nevertheless the first full-time Professor of Medicine was appointed in 1935. The appointment was conditional on the General Hospital, where the appointee was an assistant physician, raising no objection. At first the Hospital did object, but finally agreed. In order to find the salary of the Professor the University arranged that he should carry out clinical work for the City Education Committee and for the City Health Committee, for each of which he received separate remuneration. In order to increase the clinical facilities for teaching a formal agreement was reached with the City Health Committee in 1932 for students to attend Southmead Hospital and since 1939 increasing use has been made of this so that it now houses parts of the Professorial Units of Medicine, Surgery and Obstetrics. It was this that has made possible the expansion of the medical intake from less than 40 a year in 1939 to over 130 now.

At the end of the last war full time clinical chairs became the established policy of the University and in 1946 when Professor Milnes Walker was appointed to the Chair of Surgery, the Board of the Royal Hospital agreed that in future all University appointments in clinical subjects should *ipso facto* carry with them full membership of the medical staff of the Royal Hospital. The advent of the National Health Service in 1948 largely resolved – at least in theory – any remaining problems between the University and the hospitals. The Bristol Royal Hospital, the Children's Hospital, the Eye Hospital, and the Maternity Hospital were grouped together as the United Bristol Hospitals – the teaching hospital. The National Health Service Act of 1946 laid down that it is one of the duties of a teaching hospital 'to provide for the University with which the hospital is associated such facilities as appear to the Minister to be required for clinical teaching and research.'

Some of the more distinguished members of the Medical School in the early years of this century were Patrick Watson Williams, Carey Coombs and Hey Groves. Patrick Watson Williams was appointed assistant physician to the Royal Infirmary in 1888. Becoming increasingly interested in diseases of the ear, nose and throat, he resigned as physician in 1905 and was appointed the first ear, nose and throat consultant. He was one of the founders of the specialty of oto-rhino-laryngology and his work gained him international renown.

Carey Coombs entered the Bristol Medical School as a student in 1896, but moved to St. Mary's. He returned to Bristol and was appointed Physician to the General Hospital. He devoted most of his life to the study of acute rheumatism and rheumatic heart disease. His book on rheumatic heart disease is till regarded as a classic.

Hey Groves started in general practice in Kingswood where he ran a surgical nursing home with his wife as matron. From this beginning he became Surgeon to the General Hospital, Professor of Surgery, and Vice-President of the Royal College of Surgeons. He was the virtual founder of the *British Journal of Surgery* and was for many years its Editorial Secretary.

Increasing numbers of students necessitated more accommodation for the pre-clinical departments and a new medical school building. The first part of this was occupied in 1966, since when it has been gradually extended.

It can, I suggest, be claimed that the school which developed from small and tentative beginnings in the eighteenth century is certainly flourishing, and judging by the number of would-be students applying for for admission, it has become one of the most popular schools in the country.

Note on Sources

This lecture was based primarily on a study of the Minutes of the Bristol Medical School, the Minutes of the Council of University College, Bristol and the Minutes of the Council of the University of Bristol.

There is some useful material in A. Prichard, 'Early History of the Bristol Medical School', *Bristol Med Chi Journal*, x (1982); W.H. Harsant, 'Medical Bristol in the Eighteenth Century', *ibid.* xvii (1899); F. Richardson Cross, 'Early Medical Teaching in Bristol', *ibid.* xliv (1927); G. Parker in *Schola Medicinae Bristol*, John Wright & Sons, Bristol 1933.